Redemptive Yoga: A Biblical Meditation

by Amber Stowe

Redemptive Yoga: A Biblical Meditation by Amber Stowe

Text and cover photograph copyright © 2020 by Amber Stowe

All rights reserved. No portion of this book may be reproduced in any form without permission in writing from the publisher, except as permitted by U.S. copyright law, or for reviewers, who may quote brief passages in a review.

For permissions contact write.amber.stowe@gmail.com
www.amberstowe.com

ISBN# 978-1-7324237-4-9

Printed and bound by IngramSpark in the United States of America

For my graduating students, especially my goddaughter, may you always know His truth and love as you decide who you are and who you want to be.

For my two inspirational Sarahs, thank you for fighting for people's health and souls.

And thank you always to my family and friends who support and challenge me. You are loved and appreciated.

Preface

I didn't expect to learn that lesson. My heart still pounding from the climb, the sunlight glittering off the lake, the wind gently smoothing away sweat… and I thought "that was so authentic and easy." On a trip of a lifetime, traveling through Israel, our group took the morning to hike Mount Arbel. This mountain next to the sea of Galilee doesn't only have a breathtaking view. It was the mountain that rabbis would traditionally climb when they wanted to pray, away from the crowds. There is a strong likelihood Mount Arbel is where Jesus "went out on a mountainside by himself to pray" (Matthew 14:22).

The long four hour journey was one of silence and contemplation. It still stands out as one of the most fruitful and peaceful moments of prayer and connection to God I've experienced. Modern, Western views divide individuals up into separate compartments: life's various roles; emotional vs. mental vs. physical states of being; our heads vs. our hearts. Not so in ancient times. When the Shema, or greatest commandment, says to "love the Lord your God with all your heart and with all your soul and with all your mind and with all your strength", it wasn't four separate parts of a person (Mark 12:30). You were just you. All attributes and aspects were combined into one understanding of a person. They could not be separated. So as I climbed this mountain quietly, my mind wandered back and forth, from the physical task at hand to concerns and questions to God and life…and slowly they all merged and settled into peace and contemplation. The very act of physical exertion alongside of spiritual focus towards my savior worked together. Prayer had rarely felt so powerful.

It has been difficult to duplicate. Not often can one find several hours of silence; a mom of young children and a social individual, hiking quietly is as rare as showering by myself. It is one reason why I enjoy yoga among other exercise. An hour, or more, of expected pause and quiet while the body stretches, balances, and builds strength.

But it has been missing something. It has never refreshed my soul in the same way the hike did that day. So I started to try and come to class with a verse to contemplate. One day my daughter came home from kindergarten and had learned a few yoga moves herself in physical education. Then I saw a picture of my two year old son learning poses in his day care. I was struck each time by the realization that yoga has become mainstream.

Individuals from various spiritual backgrounds have different responses towards yoga. Some love it. Some simply accept it. Some have grave and valid concerns about its impact spiritually. Some discuss the different spiritual feelings they sense depending on the studio, instructor, or overall atmosphere. That being said, if there is one thing I see over and over about God's character, it is that redemption is real and alive. The Holy Spirit seeks to reach into every corner of our lives. If so, then why not yoga?

This meditative yoga is an attempt to offer such an opportunity. All truth and goodness belong to God. In most yoga studios, practitioners are asked to set an intention for class. This book hopes to set a holy intention. A time not to empty our minds but fill them with the truth and love of Jesus Christ.

If you regularly practice yoga, ask the Holy Spirit to renew you and speak to you. May this simply structured set of scriptures add value, truth, and goodness to your yoga practice; may it be one more space where a good Father redeems time; may it help you focus on His absolute deep, active, and involved love for you.

In our increasingly busy world, "May the God of hope fill you with all joy and peace as you trust in him, so that you may overflow with hope by the power of the Holy Spirit" (Romans 15:13).

Your Personal Preface:

Take some time before you begin to write your intentions, desires, and thoughts below. What made you choose this book? What do you hope it will bring to your life? What questions lie within you?

A Mini How To

Accompanying each pose, you will see three separate sets of verses. Each one attempts to emphasize a different feeling or focus during your workout—the *first set remembers God's holiness*, **the second potential reflection and encouragement**, and the third personal action. Bible verses selected are from the NIV or NASB translation.

You may want to memorize the entire verse or highlight key phrases before beginning to focus and repeat (some verses are longer to provide context). Feel free to write in your own set of verses in page margins. Your pace. Your flow. Whatever you choose, draw near to Him.

Be patient with yourself. Just as with building strength, balance, and flexibility, it takes time, dedication, and perseverance to choose to memorize scripture. The selected verses try to connect to the name or feel of the movement; this was done purposefully to connect memory. Also keep in mind that the selection of poses are the most basic that appear somewhere in most sequences. If you choose to add additional poses individually, simply carry the previous verse into your next pose or choose your own and write it in.

Over time, as you grow and practice, reciting God's word will hopefully come naturally with each pose. Instead of emptying your mind, fill it with God's truth and love. As David said in Psalm 119:11, "I have hidden your word in my heart that I might not sin against you."

Remember, "You are the light of the world. A city on a hill cannot be hidden. Neither do people light a lamp and put it under a bowl. Instead they put it on it's stand, and it give slight to everyone in the house" (Matthew 5:14-16). May the true Beginning and End of all fill you with light so you may pass that light on to a world who needs Jesus.

A Last, Thoughtful Author's Note

People that I love, admire, and respect have strong opinions on both sides regarding the pairing of Biblical scripture with yoga because of yoga's historical origins in Hinduism. Some believe there are no ties to spiritual realities as God is the owner of truth and others believe one cannot separate yoga from its original intentions to honor false gods. Some simply ask where yoga falls along the line of questioning what is permissible vs. what is beneficial. And both point to Paul's discussion in 1 Corinthians 8 to support their personal conviction.

So I must say this: this book is only for some people. Like all decisions in life, it is imperative that you listen to God's Holy Spirit during this process to determine if it is right for you individually.

If the Spirit says no, listen.

If it says yes, then move forward, making every thought captive to Christ.

Either way, be well friends.

Shavasana

Each on an adjacent plot,
our heads lie heavy. Arms and legs
splay wide and shoulders melt like butter.
We dismiss intrusive thoughts:
biopsies, broken shutters,
interest rates and aging eggs.

We die to each anxiety
and feel our hearts' soft thrum.
We watch our bellies rise and fall
buoyed by breathing. Silently
we wiggle, roll our spines, sit tall,
reborn to life's sure, holy hum.

—Susan Delaney Spear, Amethyst Review

Pre-flow: create the right intention
"Set your mind on things above" (Colossians 3:2)

Choose a verse from below or write in your favorites. Spend some time before your practice thinking on one.

1 John 4:18—There is no fear in love. But perfect love drives out fear, because fear has to do with punishment. The one who fears is not made perfect in love.

Revelation 4:11—You are worthy, our Lord and God, to receive glory and honor and power, for you created all things, and by your will they were created and have their being.

Matthew 6:25-27—Therefore I tell you, do not worry about your life, what you will eat or drink; or about your body, what you will wear. Is not life more than food, and the body more than clothes? 26 Look at the birds of the air; they do not sow or reap or store away in barns, and yet your heavenly Father feeds them. Are you not much more valuable than they? 27 Can any one of you by worrying add a single hour to your life?

James 1:5—If any of you lacks wisdom, you should ask God, who gives generously to all without finding fault, and it will be given to you.

Isaiah 26:3—You will keep in perfect peace those whose minds are steadfast, because they trust in you.

Luke 10:27—"Love the Lord your God with all your heart and with all your soul and with all your strength and with all your mind"; and, "love your neighbor as yourself."

CHILDS POSE

James 4:10
Humble yourselves before the Lord, and he will lift you up.

Philippians 4:6-7
Do not be anxious about anything, but in every situation, by prayer and petition, with thanksgiving, present your requests to God. And the peace of God, which transcends all understanding, will guard your hearts and minds in Christ Jesus.

Micah 6:8
He has shown you, O man, what is good.
And what does the LORD require of you?
To act justly and to love mercy
and to walk humbly with your God.

CAT COW

Psalm 16:7-8:
I will praise the LORD, who counsels me; even at night my heart instructs me. 8 I keep my eyes always on the LORD. With him at my right hand, I will not be shaken.

Isaiah 42:3-4
A bruised reed he will not break, and a smoldering wick he will not snuff out. In faithfulness he will bring forth justice; he will not falter or be discouraged till he establishes justice on earth. In his teaching the islands will put their hope.

Psalm 105:4
Look to the LORD and his strength; seek his face always.

DOWNWARD DOG

The pairing of these poses vary in length of time, focus, and placement within one's practice. Choose what best fits.

Psalm 11:7
*The LORD is righteous, he loves justice;
the upright will see his face.*

2 Samuel 22:29
**You, LORD, are my lamp;
the LORD turns my darkness into light.**

Psalm 34:8
Taste and see that the LORD is good;
blessed the one who takes refuge in him.

UPWARD DOG - CHATURUNGA

Revelation 4:8
*Each of the four living creatures had six wings and was
covered with eyes all around, even under its wings.
Day and night they never stop saying:
Holy, holy, holy is the Lord God Almighty,
who was, and is, and is to come.*

Psalm 68:19
**Praise be to the Lord, to God our Savior,
who daily bears our burdens.**

Psalm 147:5
Great is our Lord and mighty in power;
his understanding has no limit.

MOUNTAIN POSE

Psalm 36:6-7
Your righteousness is like the highest mountains, your justice like the great deep. You, LORD, preserve both people and animals.
7 How priceless is your unfailing love, O God!
People take refuge in the shadow of your wings.

Psalm 121:1-2
I lift up my eyes to the mountains— where does my help come from? 2 My help comes from the LORD, the Maker of heaven and earth.

1 Corinthians 16:13
Be on your guard; stand firm in the faith; be courageous; be strong.

CRESCENT MOON POSE

Psalm 19:1-4
The heavens declare the glory of God;
the skies proclaim the work of his hands.
2 Day after day they pour forth speech;
night after night they reveal knowledge.
3 They have no speech, they use no words;
no sound is heard from them.
4 Yet their voice goes out into all the earth,
their words to the ends of the world.

Psalm 148:1-3
Praise the LORD. Praise the LORD from the heavens; praise him in the heights above. 2 Praise him, all his angels; praise him, all his heavenly hosts. 3 Praise him, sun and moon; praise him, all you shining stars.

Psalm 8:3-9
3 When I consider your heavens, the work of your fingers,
the moon and the stars, which you have set in place,
4 what is mankind that you are mindful of them,
human beings that you care for them?
5 You have made them a little lower than the angels
and crowned them with glory and honor.
6 You made them rulers over the works of your hands;
you put everything under their feet:
7 all flocks and herds, and the animals of the wild,
8 the birds in the sky, and the fish in the sea,
all that swim the paths of the seas.
9 LORD, our Lord, how majestic is your name in all the earth!

FORWARD FOLD

1 Chronicles 16:11
Look to the LORD and his strength; seek his face always.

Proverbs 3:5-6
**Trust in the LORD with all your heart
and lean not on your own understanding;
6 in all your ways submit to him,
and he will make your paths straight.**

Philippians 3:12-14
Not that I have already obtained all this, or have already arrived at my goal, but I press on to take hold of that for which Christ Jesus took hold of me. 13 Brothers and sisters, I do not consider myself yet to have taken hold of it. But one thing I do:
Forgetting what is behind and straining toward what is ahead, 14 I press on toward the goal to win the prize for which God has called me heavenward in Christ Jesus.

CHAIR POSE

Revelation 20:11
Then I saw a great white throne and he who was seated on it. The earth and the heavens fled from his presence and there was no place for them.

Hebrews 4:16
Let us then approach God'd throne of grace with confidence, so that we may receive mercy and find grace to help us in our time of need.

Isaiah 6:1-3
...I saw the Lord, high and exalted, seated on the throne; and the train of his robe filled the temple. Above him were seraphim, each with six wings: With two wings they covered their faces, with two they covered their feet, and with two they were flying. 3 And they were calling to one another "Holy holy holy is the LORD almighty; the whole earth is filled with his glory."

WARRIOR 1

Exodus 15:3
*The LORD is a warrior;
the LORD is his name.*

Micah 7:7-8
But as for me, I watch in hope for the LORD, I wait for God my Savior; my God will hear me. 8 Do not gloat over me, my enemy! Though I have fallen, I will rise. Though I sit in darkness, the LORD will be my light.

Ephesians 6:10-13
Finally, be strong in the Lord and in his mighty power. 11 Put on the full armor of God, so that you can take your stand against the devil's schemes. 12 For our struggle is not against flesh and blood, but against the rulers, against the authorities, against the powers of this dark world and against the spiritual forces of evil in the heavenly realms. 13 Therefore put on the full armor of God, so that when the day of evil comes, you may be able to stand your ground, and after you have done everything, to stand.

WARRIOR 2

Zephaniah 3:17
*The LORD your God is with you,
the Mighty Warrior who saves.
He will take great delight in you;
in his love he will no longer rebuke you,
but will rejoice over you with singing.*

Romans 8:31-39
What, then, shall we say in response to these things? If God is for us, who can be against us? 32 He who did not spare his own Son, but gave him up for us all—how will he not also, along with him, graciously give us all things?

Ephesians 6:18-20
And pray in the Spirit on all occasions with all kinds of prayers and requests. With this in mind, be alert and always keep on praying for all the Lord's people. 19 Pray also for me, that whenever I speak, words may be given me so that I will fearlessly make known the mystery of the gospel, 20 for which I am an ambassador in chains. Pray that I may declare it fearlessly, as I should.

EXTENDED SIDE ANGLE/ TRIANGLE

Ephesians 1:17
I keep asking that the God of our Lord Jesus Christ, the glorious Father, may give you the Spirit of wisdom and revelation, so that you may know him better.

John 14:26-27
But the Advocate, the Holy Spirit, whom the Father will send in my name, will teach you all things and will remind you of everything I have said to you. Peace I leave with you; my peace I give you. I do not give to you as the world gives. Do not let your hearts be troubled and do not be afraid.

Matthew 28:19-20
Therefore go and make disciples of all nations, baptizing them in the name of the Father and of the Son and of the Holy Spirit, and teaching them to obey everything i have commanded you.

STAR

1 Timothy 1:17
Now to the King eternal, immortal, invisible, the only God, be honor and glory forever and ever. Amen

1 John 5:11
And this is the testimony: God has given us eternal life, and this life is in His Son.

Job 38:4
Where were you when I laid the earth's foundation?
Tell me, if you understand.

TREE POSE

Isaiah 44:3-4
*For I will pour water on the thirsty land,
and streams on the dry ground;
I will pour out my Spirit on your offspring,
and my blessing on your descendants.
4 They will spring up like grass in a meadow,
like poplar trees by flowing streams.*

Jeremiah 17:8
For he will be like a tree planted by the water, that extends its roots by a stream and will not fear when the heat comes; But its leaves will be green, and it will not be anxious in a year of drought. Nor cease to yield fruit.

Psalm 52:8-9
But I am like an olive tree
flourishing in the house of God;
I trust in God's unfailing love forever and ever.
9 For what you have done I will always praise you
in the presence of your faithful people.
And I will hope in your name,
for your name is good.

EAGLE POSE

Psalm 103:1-5
*1 praise the LORD, my soul; all my inmost being,
praise his holy name.
2 Praise the LORD, my soul,
and forget not all his benefits—
3 who forgives all your sins
and heals all your diseases,
4 who redeems your life from the pit
and crowns you with love and compassion,
5 who satisfies your desires with good things
so that your youth is renewed like the eagle's.*

Isaiah 40:3-31
**Even youths grow tired and weary, and young men stumble and fall; but those who hope in the Lord will renew their strength.
They will soar on wings like eagles;
they will run and not grow weary,
they will walk and not be faint.**

Exodus 19:4-6
You yourselves have seen what I did to Egypt, and how I carried you on eagles' wings and brought you to myself. Now if you obey me fully and keep my covenant, then out of all the nations you will be my treasured possession. Although the whole earth is mine,
you will be for me a kingdom of priests and a holy nation...

DANCER POSE

Psalm 149:3-5
*Let them praise his name with dancing
and make music to him with timbrel and harp.
4 For the LORD takes delight in his people;
he crowns the humble with victory.
5 Let his faithful people rejoice in this honor
and sing for joy on their beds.*

Jeremiah 31:4
**I will build you up again, and you, Virgin Israel, will be rebuilt.
Again you will take up your timbrels
and go out to dance with the joyful.**

Psalm 30:11-12
You turned my wailing into dancing;
you removed my sackcloth and clothed me with joy,
that my heart may sing your praises and not be silent.
LORD my God, I will praise you forever.

BOAT POSE

Isaiah 12:3
With joy you will draw water from the wells of salvation.

Isaiah 43:2
**When you pass through the waters,
I will be with you;
and when you pass through the rivers,
they will not sweep over you.**

Isaiah 49:10
They will neither hunger nor thirst,
nor will the desert heat or the sun beat down on them.
He who has compassion on them will guide them
and lead them beside springs of water.

COBRA POSE

Genesis 3:14
So the LORD God said to the serpent, "Because you have done this, Cursed are you above all livestock and all wild animals! You will crawl on your belly and you will eat dust all the days of your life."

Luke 11:9-13
So I say to you: Ask and it will be given to you; seek and you will find; knock and the door will be opened to you.
10 For everyone who asks receives; the one who seeks finds; and to the one who knocks, the door will be opened.
11 Which of you fathers, if your son asks for a fish, will give him a snake instead? 12 Or if he asks for an egg, will give him a scorpion? 13 If you then, though you are evil, know how to give good gifts to your children, how much more will your Father in heaven give the Holy Spirit to those who ask him!

Matthew 10:16
I am sending you out like sheep among wolves.
Therefore be as shrewd as snakes and as innocent as doves.

FIGURE FOUR/ PIGEON POSE

Psalm 4:8
*In peace I will lie down and sleep,
for you alone, LORD, make me dwell in safety.*

Matthew 11:28
**Come to me, all you who are weary and burdened,
and I will give you rest.**

Psalm 37:7-8
Be still before the LORD and wait patiently for him;
do not fret when people succeed in their ways,
when they carry out their wicked schemes.
8 Refrain from anger and turn from wrath;
do not fret—it only leads to evil.

CAMEL - OPEN HEART POSE

Psalm 34:18
*The Lord is close to the brokenhearted
and saves those who are crushed in spirit.*

Proverbs 3:5
**Trust in the LORD with all your heart
and lean not on your own understanding.**

Psalm 51:10
Create in me a pure heart, O God,
and renew a steadfast spirit within me.

BRIDGE POSE

John 14:6-7
Jesus answered, "I am the way and the truth and the life. No one comes to the Father except through me. 7 If you really know me, you will know my Father as well. From now on, you do know him and have seen him."

John 14:15-18
If you love me, keep my commands. And I will ask the Father, and he will give you another advocate to help you and be with you forever—17 the Spirit of truth. The world cannot accept him, because it neither sees him nor knows him. But you know him, for he lives with you and will be in you. 18 I will not leave you as orphans; I will come to you.

Ephesians 2:10
For we are God's handiwork, created in Christ Jesus to do good works, which God prepared in advance for us to do.

HAPPY BABY POSE

Psalm 139:13-14
For you created my inmost being; you knit me together in my mother's womb. 14 I praise you because I am fearfully and wonderfully made; your works are wonderful, I know that full well.

Luke 18:16
**But Jesus called the children to him and said,
"Let the little children come to me, and do not hinder them, for the kingdom of God belongs to such as these."**

Deuteronomy 6:6-7
These commandments that I give you today are to be on your hearts. 7 Impress them on your children. Talk about them when you sit at home and when you walk along the road, when you lie down and when you get up.

SUPINE TWIST / WIND RELIEVING

Ecclesiastes 7:13-15
Consider what God has done: Who can straighten what he has made crooked? When times are good, be happy but when times are bad, consider this: God has made the one as well as the other. Therefore, no one can discover anything about their future.

John 3:5
Jesus answered, "Very truly I tell you, no one can enter the kingdom of God unless they are born of water and the Spirit. 6 Flesh gives birth to flesh, but the Spirit gives birth to spirit. 7 You should not be surprised at my saying, 'You must be born again.' 8 The wind blows wherever it pleases. You hear its sound, but you cannot tell where it comes from or where it is going. So it is with everyone born of the Spirit."

James 3:3-5
When we put bits into the mouths of horses to make them obey us, we can turn the whole animal. 4 Or take ships as an example. Although they are so large and are driven by strong winds, they are steered by a very small rudder wherever the pilot wants to go. 5 Likewise, the tongue is a small part of the body, but it makes great boasts. Consider what a great forest is set on fire by a small spark.

CORPSE/SHAVASANA

Ecclesiastes 3:11-14
He has made everything beautiful in its time. He has also set eternity in the human heart; yet no one can fathom what God has done from beginning to end. 12 I know that there is nothing better for people than to be happy and to do good while they live. 13 That each of them may eat and drink, and find satisfaction in all their toil—this is the gift of God. 14 I know that everything God does will endure forever; nothing can be added to it and nothing taken from it. God does it so that people will fear him.

Romans 8:38-39
For I am convinced that neither death nor life, neither angels nor demons, neither the present nor the future, nor any powers, 39 neither height nor depth, nor anything else in all creation, will be able to separate us from the love of God that is in Christ Jesus our Lord.

Philippians 4:8
Finally, brothers and sisters, whatever is true, whatever is noble, whatever is right, whatever is pure, whatever is lovely, whatever is admirable—if anything is excellent or praiseworthy—think about such things.

***Rest now and reflect. There is an additional page at the end if you would like to journal after your work out.**

Psalm 103:13-19
As a father has compassion on his children,
so the LORD has compassion on those who fear him;
14 for he knows how we are formed,
he remembers that we are dust.
15 The life of mortals is like grass,
they flourish like a flower of the field;
16 the wind blows over it and it is gone,
and its place remembers it no more.
17 But from everlasting to everlasting
the LORD's love is with those who fear him,
and his righteousness with their children's children—
18 with those who keep his covenant
and remember to obey his precepts.
19 The LORD has established his throne in heaven,
and his kingdom rules over all.

Bank of Additional Verses

To honor those who gave me feedback about the book, I've included a wider array of verses that include even more aspects of God's character, encouragement, admonishment, topics applicable at different life stages, and other personal favorites.

1 Corinthians 6:19—Do you not know that your bodies are temples of the Holy Spirit, who is in you, whom you have received from God? You are not your own; 20 you were bought at a price. Therefore honor God with your bodies.

Psalm 90:2—Before the mountains were born or you brought forth the whole world, from everlasting to everlasting you are God.

Matthew 4:10—Jesus said to him, "Away from me, Satan! For it is written: 'Worship the Lord your God, and serve him only.'"

Ephesians 2:8-9—For it is by grace you have been saved, through faith—and this is not from yourselves, it is the gift of God— 9 not by works, so that no one can boast. 10 For we are God's handiwork, created in Christ Jesus to do good works, which God prepared in advance for us to do.

Psalm 19:8—The law of the Lord is perfect, refreshing the soul.
The statutes of the Lord are trustworthy, making wise the simple. 8 The precepts of the Lord are right, giving joy to the heart. The commands of the Lord are radiant, giving light to the eyes.

Proverbs 15:33—Wisdom's instruction is to fear the Lord,
and humility comes before honor.

Luke 18:16—But Jesus called the children to him and said, "Let the little children come to me, and do not hinder them, for the kingdom of God belongs to such as these."

Isaiah 52:7—How beautiful on the mountains are the feet of those who bring good news, who proclaim peace, who bring good tidings, who proclaim salvation, who say to Zion, "Your God reigns!"

Isaiah 54:10—"Though the mountains be shaken and the hills be removed, yet my unfailing love for you will not be shaken nor my covenant of peace be removed," says the LORD, who has compassion on you

Psalm 121:1-2—I lift up my eyes to the mountains— where does my help come from? 2 My help comes from the LORD, the Maker of heaven and earth.

Psalm 36:6-7—Your righteousness is like the highest mountains, your justice like the great deep. You, Lord, preserve both people and animals. 7 How priceless is your unfailing love, O God! People take refuge in the shadow of your wings.

Isaiah 40:22—He sits enthroned above the circle of the earth, and its people are like grasshoppers.

1 Corinthians 16:13—Be on your guard; stand firm in the faith; be courageous; be strong.

Isaiah 66:23—23 "From one New Moon to another and from one Sabbath to another, all mankind will come and bow down before me," says the Lord.

Psalm 5:7—But I, by your great love, can come into your house; in reverence I bow down toward your holy temple.

Philippians 2: 9-11—Therefore God exalted him to the highest place and gave him the name that is above every name, 10 that at the name of Jesus every knee should bow, in heaven and on earth and under the earth, 11and every tough acknowledge that Jesus Christ is Lord, to the glory of the God the Father.

Ecclesiastes 9:3-4—This is the evil in everything that happens under the sun: The same destiny overtakes all. The hearts of people, moreover, are full of evil and there is madness in their hearts while they live, and afterward they join the dead. 4 Anyone who is among the living has hope— even a live dog is better off than a dead lion!

Proverbs 26:11—As a dog returns to its vomit, so fools repeat their folly.

2 Chronicles 7: 1-3—When Solomon finished praying, fire came down from heaven and consumed the burnt offering and the sacrifices, and

the glory of the Lord filled the temple. 2 The priests could not enter the temple of the Lord because the glory of the Lord filled it. 3 When all the Israelites saw the fire coming down and the glory of the Lord above the temple, they knelt on the pavement with their faces to the ground, and they worshiped and gave thanks to the Lord, saying,"He is good; his love endures forever."

1 Timothy 6:11-12 —But you, man of God, flee from all this, and pursue righteousness, godliness, faith, love, endurance and gentleness. 12 Fight the good fight of the faith. Take hold of the eternal life to which you were called when you made your good confession in the presence of many witnesses.

Psalm 144:1—Praise be to the Lord my Rock, who trains my hands for war, my fingers for battle.

Hebrews 9:14—How much more, then, will the blood of Christ, who through the eternal Spirit offered himself unblemished to God, cleanse our consciences from acts that lead to death, so that we may serve the living God!

Ecclesiastes 11:5—As you do not know the path of the wind, or how the body is formed in a mother's womb, so you cannot understand the work of God, the Maker of all things.

Jeremiah 1:5—Before I formed you in the womb I knew you, before you were born I set you apart. I appointed you as a prophet to the nations.

Proverbs 22:6—Start children off on the way they should go, and even when they are old they will not turn from it.

Psalm 37:4—Take delight in the Lord and he will give you the desires of your heart.

Philippians 4:4—Rejoice in the Lord always. I will say it again: Rejoice!

Jeremiah 17:8—"For he will be like a tree planted by the water that sends out its roots by the stream. It does not fear when the heat comes; its leaves are always green. It has no worries in a year of drought and never fails to bear fruit.

Acts 5:30—The God of our fathers raised up Jesus, whom you had put to death by hanging Him on a cross.

Proverbs 11:30—The fruit of the righteous is a tree of life, and he who is wise saves lives.

2 Samuel 6:14—Wearing a linen ephod, David was dancing before the Lord with all his might.

Matthew 26:21—For where your treasure is, there your heart will be also.

Psalm 19:14—May these words of my mouth and this meditation of my heart be pleasing in your sight, LORD, my rock and my Redeemer.

Jeremiah 29:13—You will seek me and find me when you seek me with all your heart.

Psalm 16:11—You make known to me the path of life; you will fill me with joy in your presence, with eternal pleasures at your right hand.

Job 17:9—Nevertheless, the righteous will hold to their ways, and those with clean hands will grow stronger.

Genesis 1:1—In the beginning, God created the heavens and the earth.

Psalm 119:89—Forever, O LORD, Your word is settled in heaven.

Jeremiah 23:23-24—"Am I only a God nearby," declares the LORD, "and not a god far away? Who can hide in secret places so that I cannot see them?" declares the LORD. "Do not I fill heaven and earth?" decades the LORD.

John 16:33—I have told you these things, so that in me you may have peace. In this world you will have trouble. But take heart! I have overcome the world.

Isaiah 59: 1-2—Surely the arm of the Lord is not too short to save, nor his ear too dull to hear. 2 But your iniquities have separated you from your God; your sins have hidden his face from you so that he will not hear.

Reflection Space

Take time here to write any reflections, realizations, or moments of conviction, joy, peace, etc. How did God meet you on your mat or in life today?

www.ingramcontent.com/pod-product-compliance
Lightning Source LLC
Chambersburg PA
CBHW071506080526
44587CB00016B/2711